Contents

Development of Biorhythm

In order for the human body to keep up with the day to day activities and to also keep on existing, there is the need for the body to be controlled or regulated by an internal factor. This factor is responsible for our behavioral pattern in general. It regulates our body systems to response of different conditions.

We are not all the same. Our body system reacts differently to different conditions for example, a man that is very physically active in the evening, might not be, during the day time or the reverse could be the case. Someone might be uncomfortable or fall sick in summer but energetic in winter.

Biorhythms have started for as long as 3,000 years ago, when the scientists of ancient Greece record regularly, the basic bodily functions such as, the female menstrual cycle, pulse rate, and respiration. These regular records made them come to a notice that there are both Good and bad days in man which controls their behavioral pattern.

But the theory of biorhythm was developed in Berlin by Wilhelm fliess an otolaryngologist, a patient of Sigmund Freud and president of the German Academy of Sciences in the 19th century .William fliess undertook various research and became convinced that the 23 and 28 days of biorhythm are crucial in human life which he called the 23 day period "male" and the 28 days period "female". At this time, Dr.Wilhelm fliess came about the theory that man has this internal "clock" that continues counting throughout lifetime until death, and his research contained many mathematical and statistical approach which not only confused people but pissed them off but was appealing to Sigmund Freud.

Someone who wasn't aware of fliess work, Hermann swoboda a professor at the university of Vienna aware through careful observation in mans attitude, came to conclusion with Wilhelm fliess theory that there is a certain rhythmical periodicity which affects man and his behavioral pattern through thorough and careful research so that he publishes his first two books *"periodicity in man life and "studies in the basis of psychology"*. After that, he published a booklet that contains instructions on biorhythm called *"the critical days of man"* but one of his best written or published book was titled *"the year of seven"* which contains more of mathematical theory to biorhythm approach. Also, an Estonian born researcher on biorhythm Nikolai parna published a book in German called *"Rhythm, life and creation"*.

Further research shows that each and every human being inherits a bisexual (male and female) characteristics in one way or the other.

Alfred teltscher a professor of engineering and a mathematics student claimed that, there were predetermined periods when a person possesses poor performance in intellectual pursuit, and there are periods when a high performance of intellectual pursuit could be attained. He came about this by observing a cyclic fluctuation in the intellectual capabilities of his students in the 33-day cycle.

The use of biorhythm had been neglected and abandoned for a long time because people see the method of its calculations as being complicated or not-understandable to a layman until it was simplified and revived again as a result of new research and publications on the matter.

Steadily but slowly the public started to develop an interest in the subject of biorhythms in an ergonomic manner so that they use it to reduce anticipated mistakes that might lead to accidents. Some group or association began talking on the subject even Britain had developed great interest on the subject by increased developers and researchers on the subject to the extent that people started paying a certain amount of fee for the service. So, we might want to ask - how does biorhythm affect us and our daily living?

We need to take into notice that there are three cycles of biorhythm which are, the physical cycle, emotional cycle and intellectual cycle. Some awareness of this cycles(s) will enable us know our effective time and ineffective time so that we know how to make use of it properly. Each of this rhythm plays a crucial role in human life right from the moment the brain comes to life till it dies.

When you are at your most effective period, the first half of the cycle ascends giving the (+) phase and might bring about a breakpoint called critical stage if continued for a long period. Critical stage or breakpoint as in the drastic fall in the stress level when reaching a peak. Your stress level remains at a high level until gradually, the rhythm returns to the former state of the cycle called the second half. The second phase brings in a new life force in itself (renewed strength or vigor). When the first half of the cycle gradually dies at midpoint, it revives again through the positive phase. This pattern repeats itself over and over again.

One

The Biorhythm Cycles

Like it was stated previously, there are three major stage of biorhythm cycles. The physical cycle has a duration of 23 days, the emotional cycle has a duration of 28 days and the intellectual cycle has a duration of 33 days but another rhythm which cannot be regarded as a primary one was discovered later which is called the intuitive cycle and controls the subconscious perception called the sixth sense. so, they control these three major areas of human behavior. It was said that these biorhythm cycles are a potential answer to our on and off days, and people can increase the quality of their lives by monitoring their biorhythms and acting to it accordingly. They help to indicate our potential physical ability, emotional being or intellectual capability and limitations on any particular day, they are set to zero at the moment of birth and they also have a lot to do with trigonometry.

Each cycle begins on the day our brain starts working till the day it dies that is; from birth to death and can easily be calculated with your birth date. Put at the back of your mind that one day, you shall return to that point of the cycles you were, initially at birth which is zero (All your biorhythm cycle will return to point zero). This time means death to some people and rebirth to others. Also Put in mind that in any form, this is not astrology even though they are similar in the sense that it deals with the individual and the attitude they adopt but it doesn't involve any form of magic.

Biorhythm involves calculating a physiological function and relating the results to our physiological Cycle. Also, Thommen's hypothesis claimed that he could predict the sex of a child through biorhythms during conceptions. He claims that if during conception, the mothers physical cycle (23 day "masculine") was at a high point, she's likely to give birth to a male child and if during conception, the mother's Emotional cycle (28 day "feminine") was at a high point, she's likely to give birth to a female child.

The Physical Cycle

The physical cycle which comes from our masculine inheritance, is the shortest biorhythm which last 23 days divided into (11.5 days positive and 11.5 days negative) and often represented in a red line. It is filled with a very great and impressive performance because there must be the ability for the physical to carry through task at hand for a positive result to be attained as it influences physical factors such as physical coordination, stamina, sex drive and resistance to disease.

Sometimes, the effect of the cycle is not noticeable and sometimes apparent. It starts from the moment you awake in the morning, stretch, yawn and go off to the bathroom.

The physical cycle/positive phase

The 11.5 days of the physical biorhythm cycle which is the first positive half phase, which comes to a peak above the zero point mostly around the 6th in the chart, comes with zeal on the part of the individual from the time he awakes in the morning till the time he goes back into bed. He awakens with full vital energy readily prepared for the day. He does everything with ease and this is apparent from the first time he gets out of bed - instead of the sluggish continuous yawning, and the walking tirelessly to the bathroom, he awakes in full anticipation for the day, have a nice shave, a hearty meal, and a nice drive to the office. He volunteers to do many tasks because he's virile and his bodily system won't allow him to stay idle for long. He gets actively proactive even in sports and this energy carries him throughout the rest of the day and that is why at this phase, athletes may tend to do better in sports.

Also, in this phase, the individual is resistant to diseases because their immune system will be stronger at this time around that is why biorhythm-wise surgeons, prefer to operate their patient during this phase because the operations are much more successful then. It is advisable to schedule activities requiring great physical exertion for this period too.

The physical cycle/Negative phase & critical day

Unlike the positive phase, the other half phase which is the negative phase that comes to a peak usually around the 23rd day in the chat, comes without any zeal on the part of the individual from the Time he awakens in the morning, till when he goes to bed at night. He awakens even with a feeling of tiredness after having long hours of sleep, not readily or not too prepared for the day, all he wants to do is, go back to sleep again but he has no option than to go about his daily activities. Now, everything he does seems like difficult so that he has to stress himself to do it. He goes off to bed sluggishly, yawning sleepily and walking tiredly to the bathroom, fumbling for something, maybe the shaving stick or toothbrush or whatever. If possible, he might skip shaving or brushing altogether. He does not have interest in running the day and even if he considers doing anything, he might make a mistake. All this, because he is in the period of recovery, so that the body can recoup itself for the positive phase again.

Unlike the positive phase, instead of him volunteering or offering to do tasks, he prefers to day dream, take a nap or rest. He postpones some task and delegate some duties. This lack of interest carries him throughout the day until he returns back into bed. This days are called critical days or transition days.

On this critical day, you are more likely to be exposed to danger and illness as your Body is in the stage of transition from the positive phase to the negative phase or the reverse, which brings about imbalance, so it's better to avoid physical efforts and engage only in routine task, and if you have to engage in any physical activity for example sports, make sure to eat healthily, have good rest, and exercise very well - make yourself fully prepared so that at least, you could make a difference. Reports shows that in athletes, injuries occur in critical days".

On this physical "critical days" it is advisable not to operate dangerous machines, undergo any surgeries whatsoever whether you are the surgeon or patient.

The Rhythmic pattern on physical cycle.

Everything about life, especially our body system has a reoccurring pattern. name it; the alternation of the night and day, cold and heat, summer and winter, etc. Even, everything about our existence, a sought of *"Deja-vu"*. Generally, we have biological clocks and we respond to them as they govern the functions of our body system especially our health. There are morning people and evening people, that is; some people are active during the early stage of the day and become inactive during the late hours of the day while some people might start their day sluggishly and become vibrant in the evening which is controlled by the circadian rhythm (sleep and wake cycle). All this has to do with their biological clocks. This times too, can be interlaced to each other. The morning person today, might be the evening person tomorrow and the evening person today, might be the morning person tomorrow.

Sometimes we feel like we are experiencing a dramatical change in our behavioral responses. Sometimes in the day, we feel like we are experiencing a change from the negative to positive or from positive to negative; Note: the meals we take sometimes plays part on our physiological behavior so it's necessary to have a good meal at regular intervals so that the body can maintain a steady stamina flow and also, this can be related to the circadian rhythm again. For example, in the early morning hours at about 4.00 a.m. the body temperature is at its lowest and at its highest around 4. 00p.m that same day - the reason for the swing in energy level at times.

In the negative phase of the physical cycle, occurs a strong health factor. At this phase, there is every chance for you to fall sick or a tendency to be susceptible to illness. Sometimes what you do in the (+) positive stage of the cycle might not have an adverse effect on you than when you do them in the (-) negative stage or critical stage of the cycle. Drinking heavily when in the positive phase of the cycle might not place an adverse effect on your health but can make you fall seriously sick when you are in the (-) negative phase. Definitely, it would do us good for us to take notice of biorhythm phase we fall into so that we do things in adequate manner for example drinking adequately or little in the critical stage. Also, a lack of care in all dietary manners, will affect sleeping habits. We should occasionally learn to take care in these critical times by taking moderate exercises, regular meals, and establishing routine habits in order to stand in proper position with your rhythmic pattern. Driving on an empty stomach, will lead to adverse stomach problems, lowering of blood sugar level and can in turn, lead to lack of focus on the part of the driver which might lead to accident.

Talking about the other cycle which cannot be regarded as primary (intuitive cycle), contains patterns such as, perception, psychic and success.

The Emotional Cycle

Or shall we say factors that influence feelings? The 28-day cycle which is related to the well-known menstrual cycle. Like the physical cycle, the emotional rhythm starts with a critical day. From positive to negative, its transition date starts fourteen days and ends on the third critical day then, fourteen days after that. It has a mini-critical day on day eight when going to the positive phase and at day twenty-eight when going to the negative phase. When in the negative phase, you are susceptible to different kind of emotional conditions. You are susceptible to anger, nervousness, irritability and so on.

You can also use your emotional biorhythm cycle to determine the kind of job, suitable for your personality - according to your temperament. The emotional cycle affects our spiritual being, it affects sensibility, mood, creativity, and affection.

The Emotional Cycle/Positive Phase.

Like It was stated earlier, every human being inherits a bisexual characteristic. The feminine characteristic is directly related to the emotional cycle. Wilhelm fliess defined the emotional cycle as the manifestation of the cells influencing the feminine inheritance in our make-up. In the positive phase, we tend to develop certain behaviors like, optimism, kindness, gratitude, love and confidence, passion, or elation. Then, around the eight day of this phase, we reach a peak that starts to decline into the negative phase.

The emotional phase plays an important role in our social life - the mutual day to day relationship with people. If you are a sales person, during this phase, you tend to be on a more agreeable term with your customers, in relationships you become a better lover, Public speaker tends to gain confidence even when facing a larger audience which helps in captivating the listeners but when you are in your off days you can make adequate preparation if its something you really need to do. Awareness of your emotional state puts you in the better position for moderation.

The emotional cycle/ The negative phase & critical stage.

In this phase, the recipient seems to feel gloomy and or emotionally drained. A feeling of despair, anger, sadness, hate or coldness etc. He gets moody and tends to react negatively to situations. If he was in the positive phase, he might overlook mistakes and forgive easily but here in the negative phase, he's the one looking for mistakes and error. A friend of Ms. Sarah, said something referring to another person. Ms. Sarah having overhead these words, took it personal and had to shoot back at her friend in anger only to hear that she wasn't the one her friend was referring to. A simple biorhythm application made it evident that emotionally, she was in the negative phase about to cross the critical stage.

A little challenging word from your partner might make you burst out in anger or you become unhappy, unappreciative, moody, pessimistic until you divert slowly to the positive phase again.

In this negative phase, a calmer attitude should be maintained as much as possible. Stressful activities should be avoided. Even driving may be avoided both on negative phase days and critical days.

The critical days normally start in day 1 and 14 and as well, you will suffer from mood swings in the critical stage of the emotional cycle. You might be terribly pessimistic, and short circuited to actions that might trigger your anger but depending on your temperament.

Intellectual Cycle

During the shift of the negative phase to the positive phase in the middle where the point is at its peak, we tend to be vibrant mentally- our power of perception, problem solving, reasoning ability tends to ascend. The intellectual cycle regulates a person sense of reason, concentration, memory, deduction, decision making etc.

The intellectual cycle (33 days) discovered by Alfred teltstcher and just like the name sounds, affects mental faculty which belongs to both masculine and feminine inheritance. during this period, we tend to solve problems more easily through our sub-conscious and creative ideas tend to come more easily. You become more open to challenging debates, and solving riddles. Studying at this phase helps a lot, as it makes assimilation easier.

The Intellectual Cycle/The positive phase

As human beings in general, we only utilize 35% of our mental capability. To avoid the brain from being further below capacity, it needs to be exercised on a regular basis, in fact It needs to be exercised every time. In terms of a receptive memory, we should train ourselves to remember things often for example things like dates and events, instead of constantly relying on a reminder or calendar. We need to be able to do simple calculations without the calculator but despite this, our intellectual capabilities would not let us down during this phase, as we learn and assimilate quickly, we have solid reasoning ability, and this is usually the best time to take a test or sit for an examination. For industrial workers this is the best time to operate machineries.

The Intellectual cycle/Negative phase & critical stage

During this period, the brain seems like not wanting to do much work.

The individual involved, will also experience a little decline in his mental ability. Not that anything is wrong with the brain at this stage, but let us put it as though the brain needs some rest.

Making the right decision becomes impossible, concentration becomes a problem so that you don't understand what you've been studying, there tend to be a confusion in your reasoning even conversations seems to go off-key. This occurs in the negative phase of the intellectual cycle but more apparent in the critical stage of the intellectual cycle.

Students during this period(s), in a lecture room find concentration and understanding of the subject a little or very difficult despite they love that subject. This might be because they find their minds often drifting away so that they miss vital points or they just can't get their heads to think straight. And sometimes, those who manage to concentrate seems not to understand a thing or forgets almost everything immediately after leaving the lecture room. As a student preparing for an exam, you try to study maybe hard, then finally, you sit for the anticipated examination without knowing you are in the negative or critical phase intellectually, don't be surprised as you might omit or overlook questions you are familiar with and or you've studied well for only to blame yourself for being a fool after submitting the test.

The thing about this negative phase in the intellectual cycle is that most times, it is not noticeable by its recipient. A sales person might be passing through one of this stage if he gives his customer a double change. People who often exercise their brains don't seem to notice much difference in intellect depreciation. Sometimes you try to remember a familiar name but it seems your memory had deserted you for the moment only for you to remember later through your subconscious. Sometimes you might even forget the name of your first child during this period.

Two

Biorhythm and Man

The inter-change of serial succession in the human body cell is never ending and will continue until death takes its place. This rhythm of basic serial successions like the alternation of day and night and other rhythms are the basis of changes in the human behavior for example the circadian rhythm but more importantly, the Bio-rhythm. This cyclic event surprisingly, is not noticed by the individual except for the few ones that studied biorhythms or cyclic performance in man. This concept exists as a result of the relationship between man and nature. Like the day of birth when the three biorhythm cycles came to life, a day occurs when these three cycles start and ignites again. i call this "the biorhythm ignition" or "the ignition of biorhythm". Research shows that this day occurs on 21,252 days (58 years and 62days) approximately from the date of birth- for some, this is the triple critical day after that. During this period, 925 physical cycles, 759 sensitivity cycles, and 644 intellectual cycles would have occurred. But before reaching this stage where the three cycles reach identical point, each rhythm will continue its routine process from positive to negative or negative to positive.

Under circumstances, its normal for us to have the good and

bad days some further believe in "luck days" well, that is the reason why each time we need to attend a special occasion, its best to check our biorhythm status to know in advance what we are capable of achieving. When your biorhythm is calculated and you see the proposed date as much of a discouragement, you have the choice of postponing the event if you can and it would have been so much better if teachers or lectures could put biorhythm into consideration to improve their students performance but sadly, some just had to criticize the concept of biorhythm, some even rejects it, and act ignorantly toward its usefulness. someone once said to my face "this theory cannot be relied upon" until I asked him if he had tested it to be sure of its validity. The issue of biorhythm is one that should be tested to be sure of its validity and to be sure of its validity, is to be fully informed.

The Biogram

Your personal biogram or biorhythm chart reveals your potential behavior patterns. It also can help in various health aspect like reducing obesity, reducing alcoholic obsession, improving potency and it goes hand in hand with metaphysics when it comes to health issues - responding to drug therapy.

Example of a Biogram:

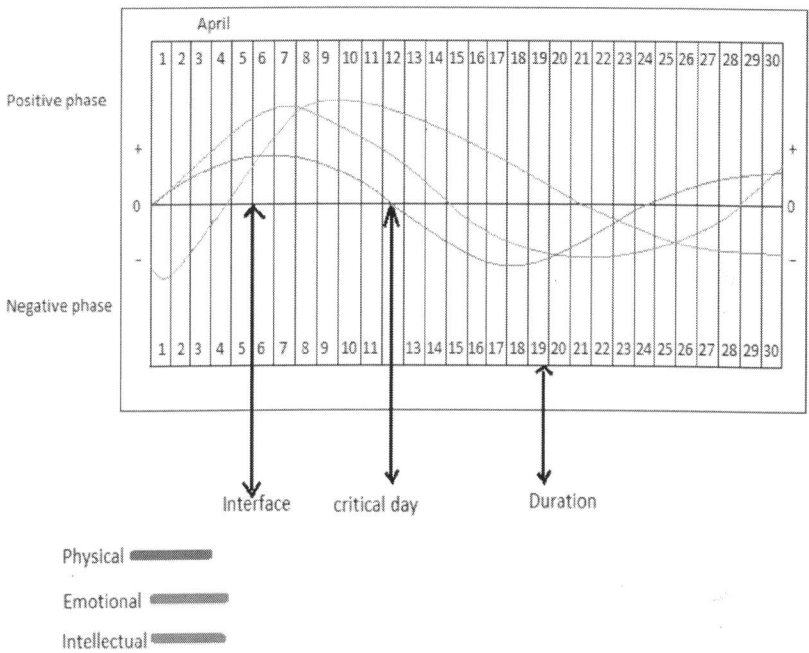

Knowing your personal rhythm through the biogram reveals a lot and can make you improve the way you live every day.

Applying the biogram to the physical phase, you will realize from the chart that, the best time to engage in any physical activity within the month would start from the 1st to 10th because at this point, you will be at the apex of your energy level but on the 12th to 24th, it would be best not to strain your energy too much. The time you should be watchful on the chart regarding the physical cycle are, 12th and 24th which are the critical days because if you are not careful on this days, physically, you could make a blunder.

Biorhythm- Human factor

Making use of Biorhythm is a factor for getting the best result in every event. Have you ever watched a football match where the ball was delivered to a well-known skilled striker only for him to kick it offside even with the goal keeper out of the goal post? Perhaps he was in the critical stage of the physical cycle, he would be better off if he monitored his biorhythm in advance before the match.

The physical rhythm relates to our muscle fibers, and everything we do with our physical ability culminates as a result of the physical rhythm. Being aware of the shift in the interface between the negative and positive rhythm, prevents you from running into majority of problems. Ignorance of the term "Biorhythm" would not allow some of us to take real consideration of our physical, emotional or intellectual state before engagement in an activity.

The regular workaholic would work his way throughout the night, fighting off sleep with a cup of coffee and self-control. Unfortunately, he doesn't know what's called biorhythm or even heard of it, so to him, its nobody's business if he fights his way to perform extra task, until later, when he realizes the next day tha what he did the previous night was total rubbish. If this fellow continues stubbornly to prolong this sleepless night, he might reach a breakdown both physically and intellectually if his biorhythm isn't in his favor within those days. Biorhythm also contributes to obesity, how? Our food intake affects the daily rhythm of adipose tissue functions present in our body clock and the way we react to sleep (if negatively- that is; sleeping deficiency), brings about metabolic disorder - causes of weight gain or diabetes.

As we all know, the body clock is responsible for our sleeping and waking pattern, hormonal regulation, temperature regulation and feeding habits. And if there happens to be any disorder with any of the above there is likely to be a vulnerability to obesity and irregularity in our body system as our physiological and psychological pattern should be in synchronization with our internal and external cycles.

- Feeding pattern: what we eat determines how our body responds to food. People who eat large meals only once in a while, are susceptible to obesity than those who eat smaller meals frequently and each meal eaten in different times of the day, has its own different effect in the body but it is observed that the most important meal of the day is the breakfast and dinner and the reasons for sleeping deficiency sometimes, has to do with eating more fast food which contains more fat, cholesterols, salt and sugar than vegetables. So, its better to eat more of vegetables and fruit rather than snacks or pork.
- Sleeping and waking pattern: people who work nights occasionally, do not know what harm they cause to their endocrine systems - causing obesity and sleeping deficiency and this is partly due to the change in eating habits. It would be advisable for one to go to bed at the same time every night so that the internal clock should readily adapt to this habit but remember this; Always switch off the lights before going to bed because it affects the sleeping and waking pattern and you know, the body as a way of responding to light.

The body clock (circadian rhythm) is worth considering when trying to exercise your muscles, arranging your training schedule in accordance with your body clock means better performance. Exercise during the day time let's say (12. 00p.m to 3. 00p.m) causes an increase in testosterone level which is vital for the muscle anabolism - consequently, this is the perfect time to exercise.

More than one occasion, there had been a consistent relationship between biorhythm and sports, even though not directly related to physical energy and there are various results, that athletes and gymnasts perform better in the positive phase. Attention to biorhythms by a coach will allow that coach to bring about better performance by the athletes not to win the game, but to motivate them to do better. It is true that biorhythms will not predict the outcome of events for you but can indicate to you your given potential for that day. its only left to you to make use of the information you get to your advantage.

Coming to the emotional cycle, if you fall into the category of the aggressive temperament, you should always try to keep on a low-key in a situation whereby you are below par rhythmically. Any slightest loose attitude by you, might not bring about a favorable outcome. everything we do is governed by irresistible rules that makes us fit into our environment, but we need to fight off impulses in order to conform with the society.

The cyclic behavior of man is different from his natural rhythm. Our behavioral pattern is as a result of our environment and getting acquainted with the rules, is understanding the change of the rhythm between the interface. That is - awareness of the good and bad days. As said by a celebrated Greek physician 3,000 years ago, that we are subjected to good and bad days irrespective of our health.

The Critical days

The day in which the cycles begins to transit from one phase to another is called a "critical day" and the day where any of the cycles is at its peak, is a mini-critical day. This days are the most important or popular aspect of biorhythm because, people believe that most dangerous occurrence happens on that day. Each critical day can be located on the biogram where any of the cycle touches the interface before shifting to the other phase *"the turning point.* This change determines on that particular day, if you would be providential or inauspicious.

Normally, a change in circumstance will always have an effect on the individual personality, a change in environment for instance. I have come across a mother whose adolescent child fell sick immediately she left him and traveled to another country for sometimes, then when she came back, that child was well again - Though this incident could be related to the relationship between mother and child, it wouldn't be wrong if we term this as change in circumstances. You plan going to an event with a friend only for her to disappoint you by going without you - your reaction would be a mixture of emotional and intellectual imbalance or after a lot of effort, sleepless nights, and a lot of research, you thought you have managed to get yourself an awesome piece of content waiting to be published but you got rejected on the way- this bad situation might and might not happen on a critical day, but your reactions to these situations would vary on different days for instance a double-critical day would mean a catastrophe.

60% of accidents that occur, are more likely on critical or double-critical days. This are days when the self is to be properly checked and caution is to be made. On this days, if careless or the self is not properly utilized, injury or accidents might occur.

Three

Biorhythm and Compatibility.

Biorhythm plays a crucial role on the agreeable pattern or relationship between individuals. Even though we as humans try hard to be in an agreeable pattern with others, sometimes might not be successful as we are naturally competitive in nature. Many times, we find faults with someone and do not want to have anything to do with them. Sometimes we feel as though we are not compatible with someone or their standard doesn't measure up to ours then, relationship with such persons comes blurred though the reverse could be the case at other times. Sometimes, you attend a party, you meet a complete stranger, then you carry conversations as though you've been friends for decades. You seem to like that person or have a certain interest for them. In this case, the both of you; your personal biorhythms are somehow in line with each other than the latter case. It might be surprising at times, when the people you predicted you won't fit together, happens to get along fine with you fine.

But i want us to first note that, if there is a difference between two partners biorhythm cycle; for example, person A is on a physical good day, while person B is on a physical bad day, it is called "biorhythm divergence". Understanding our personal biograms, should enable us know the course of action to take at a particular time, and understand that we experience different interchange of cycles at different times - even between two intimate partners. A partner might be in the mood for intimacy, while the other isn't. Knowing these simple things solves relationships incompatibility to some extent- it enables you to compare and contrast.

Compatibility and Relationships

Two people might not necessary feel the same way at the same time, intellectually, emotionally, or physically. Partner A might be physical aroused while partner B just prefers to have some rest. They just have a different interchange in the positive and negative phase physically. If Mr. A and Mr. B seems to be physically adventurous at a particular time, they can also have their physical biorhythm cycle going down the negative phase almost, or at the same time. An athlete needs to know in advance the date he would fall on the critical stage in his preferred cycle so as to make adjustments.

In the event of love making, between two intimate partners, that have different interchange of cycles, a lot of compromise needs to be made in order to make the activity a worthwhile experience. We should know that in the event of love making, the physical and emotional cycle is essential. Now, let us say, partner A is in the positive phase physically and emotionally while partner B is in the positive phase emotionally but negative physically, then partner A should be the one to guide or take control in the love making activity provided that each partner allows for the difference in the interchange and understand how this would affect their individual performance, they would get along very well together.

Between two partners, physical compatibility tends to bring physical attraction, sexual appeal and sexual satisfaction but without the emotional compatibility, which is essential in a relationship, the union is incomplete as Love is missing. Couples who falls into this category will mostly become total strangers and more of roommates after their children are grown ups and left home. But this couple are obliged to parental responsibility and cooperative when these children are young and at home.

In emotional compatibility only, this case is a little bit different.

Between this couple, there is undeniable feelings for each other but still, Love without sexual satisfaction is still incomplete. And this is the reason why so many partners seek sexual satisfaction outside marriage despite the love they have for each other.

Intellectual compatibility only, between partners is something I totally not approve of in marriages. Couples who fall into this category are those that attract their partners by impressing them. A woman might be attracted to a male because of his personality, or intelligence but this is necessary not love and which with time, that ability to continue impressing that same partner fades away.

The Emotional and physical compatibility: Despite that, this two are essential in relationships, they aren't Enough. In the case of these partners, the both of them are in love but the woman loves the most and mostly the more sentimental. The only friction in this type of relationship, is lack of knowledge, understanding and judgement between them. They do things because of their emotions but not because it is the right thing to do.

The Intellectual and Physical compatibility: This type of partners will always get a first day click. And might usually admit that they are in love because this attraction, mutual understanding and sexual satisfaction is there. A day without a conversation will be a little bit difficult. But there seems to be a friction; with time, submission by the wife will become difficult especially if there is a conflict. There are situations like this whereby each partner will expect the other to apologize first. They become too wise for themselves.

Intellectual and Emotional compatibility: This is a Platonic love. It would have been a perfect relationship, if not the absence of sex. And as a partner that they are, they would do well. Nobody understand and love their partner better than they do but that sexual part is a No-no. This type of compatibility ratings usually falls between 60-80%.

The above 80% compatibility ratings are rare, but people who fall into this category are what a perfect match should be. The mutual understanding, feelings, connection and sexual satisfaction are always there.

Every couple wants to improve their love life, every friend wants to be in good terms with one another, every working colleagues wants to have a better working relationship, every sales person wants to understand their clients better, every executive wants to understand their workers and subordinate better, every football manager wants to know the abilities of their athletes and all this can be achieved through Biorhythms and research also showed that lack of attention to employees biorhythm, is the major reason for reduction in the quality of work in administrative jobs and also, in many cases, affects executives decision making.

Some couple tend not to be in good terms with one another, some are never in agreeable terms and no matter how much they try, they never had success. Little wonder why there are so many divorced couple today. The case would have been different if every partner was aware of each other biorhythm pattern and how it affects their difference in behavior so that they can act according to the knowledge. With this knowledge, they would have more tendency to do things in common, and achieve best results. The individual chart and biogram should be calculated accordingly. But the truth about Biorhythms and compatibility lies in the fact that it does not predict the outcomeof a relationship but shows its potential.

We all seek different things in a relationship, we all look for different qualities in a person. Some might be seeking sexual relationships, some working relationships, some mutual relationships. And in every marriage, we all seek different qualities in a partner. Face, it, some will settle for a sought of bad guy, some a good guy, and some a sex maniac. You see, the fact that your potential partner has a 99%-compatible rating with you, doesn't mean they will totally be like you- That is a danger sign and believe it no relationship is ever perfect and believe it again, no matter how sweet a relationship might seem, we would always want a little bitterness.

The way in which biorhythm is best used is, as an instrument for determining the person suitable for what you would need in a partner. A 100% compatibility in a relationship is useless if you don't find that spot you need in a partner, to fit into your standard or can suit your goals. For the person looking for the sexual aspect in a partner, a 96% compatibility will be useless if only the physical compatibility is below par to his standard.

What if you are married already, and not compatible? The way out is that, both partners should understand the areas they are compatible and focus building on that area or like I said earlier, " can make compromises" nevertheless, a full compatibility in rare cases doesn't guarantee a successful marriage.

Compatibility as A Team

The same way two partners need to get along with each other very well, in accordance with bio rhythmic cycles, so as it is necessary for a team of persons. In every organization, a team will do better, and be in harmony with themselves, when they work in accordance with their biorhythm status.

For the football coach who is trying to figure out which player to use at a particular time, the biogram table can be of help.

The Biogram Table

Day(s)	0	1	2	3	4	5	6	7	8	9	10	x	33	32	31	30	29	28	27	26	25	24	23	22	21	20	19	18	17	16	15	14	13	12	11
Physical Cycle (%)	100	91	83	74	65	57	48	39	30	22	13	.	-	-	-	.	-	.	.	-	.	.	100	91	83	74	65	57	48	39	30	22	13	4	4
Emotional Cycle (%)	100	93	86	79	71	64	57	50	43	36	29	.	-	.	-	.	.	100	93	86	79	71	64	57	50	43	36	29	21	14	7	.	7	14	21
Intellectual Cycle (%)	100	94	88	82	76	70	64	58	52	46	39	-	100	94	88	82	76	70	64	58	52	46	39	33	27	21	15	9	3	3	9	15	21	27	33

Comparison and Contrast in Compatibility

Jim and Benjamin are both workers in an organization. They got employed the same day in the same department and from the very day they've got to know each other, they've built a strong bond. They had talks on various subjects and behaved more like brothers. Come around when these two are together, and you would think its another world of friendliness in itself and whenever they are not around, you would think the office is a deserted monks cave. These two have been very good friends from the scratch and it is obvious they share common interest except for the difference that, one seems to be more industrious than the other. Using their birth date to check their biorhythm for a particular month, this is what it looks like;

MR. Jim

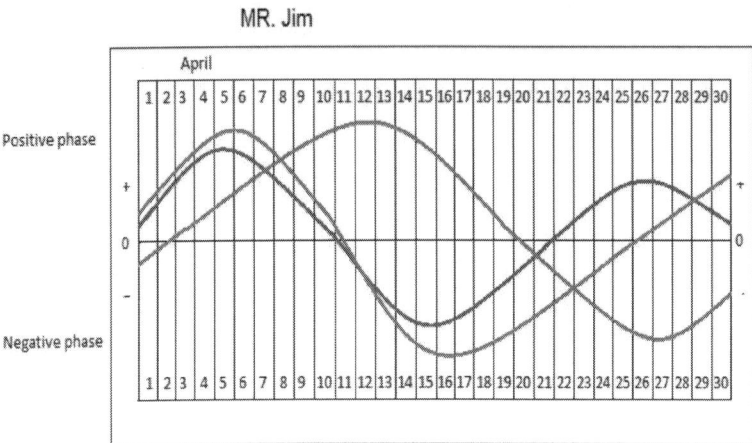

MR. Benjamin

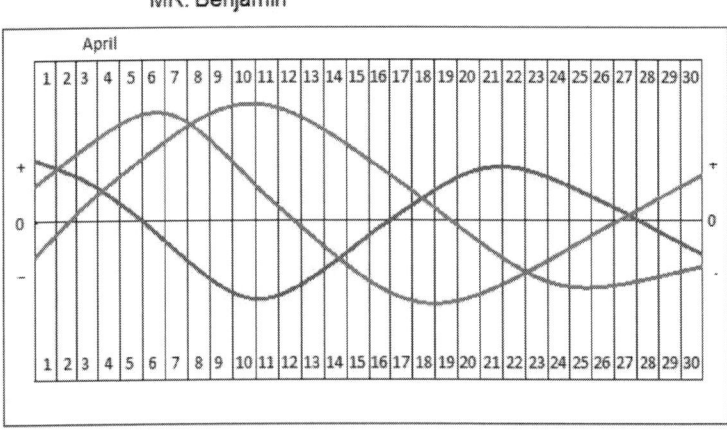

From the biogram above, you will notice that;

Physically

Mr. Jim and Mr. Benjamin cycle are obviously opposite physically. In Mr. Ben's case, the cycle transits from the positive to the negative on the 5th, where he first hit a critical day that month (this day must have been a terrible day physically for Mr. Ben) then on the 16th when he went up the positive phase and transited back to the negative phase on 27th. So, his critical days for that month are, on the 5th, 16th and 27th respectively.

But Mr. Jim's critical day started on the 11th of that month where he was descending bio rhythmically from the positive phase to the negative phase then, on the 21st when he was ascending to the positive phase.

On the 1st of April in that year, Mr. Jim was on the second day of his physical rhythm and Mr. Benjamin was on the seventh day of his physical rhythm the difference between both rhythms is Five, relating that figure to the biogram table, gives us a compatibility rating of 57%

Emotionally

Mr. Jim's and Mr. Benjamin's emotional rhythm are almost the same. Mr. Jim hit a critical day on the 11th and Mr. Benjamin hit a critical day on the 12th both going to the negative phase. Towards the positive phase, Mr. Jim had a critical day on the 26th and Mr. Benjamin had a critical day on the 27th. It is evident that they are only one day different in this rhythm.

On the first of that month, Mr. Jim is on the 5th day of the emotional rhythm, and Mr. Benjamin is on the 4th day of the emotional rhythm. The difference between both rhythm is only one and the compatibility rating is 93%

Intellectual

Mr. Jim and Mr. Benjamin's intellectual rhythm is what I would call almost the same thing. they both had a critical day on the 2nd and 19th and in the same pattern.

On the first day of that month, Mr. Jim is on the 16th day of the rhythm so as Mr. Benjamin. The difference is 0 and the compatibility rating is 100%

Four

Simple calculations To

Biorhythms.

The past times problem of establishing or determining biorhythms have been solved to a remarkable extent, as there are so many apps all over the web that offers free biorhythm calculations. The web had solved the problems of long complaints that the biorhythm calculations are hard to come by however, these calculations had also been brought down to its simplest form, so that anybody can do it without much ado.

From time to time, there have been different approach to biorhythm calculations, and each biorhythm specialist, seems to have different methods of dealing with them. Through the color codes of each cycle, you should well be able to plot the chart and differentiate each cycle - red for the physical cycle, blue for the emotional cycle and green for the intellectual cycle.

The Biorhythm can be calculated by, dividing the numbers of days (leap year included) lived by the three cyclic periods. Which can be calculated in decimals or fractions, depending on your choice, where the 23 and 28 days cycle repeats every 644 days and the 23, 28 and 33 days cycle repeats every 21,252 days.

All Biorhythm charts are the same with the exception of the difference in its rhythmical transition. But this table below will also aid you in calculating the biorhythm without a calculator.

though the calculations are borrowed:

DAYS	1	2	3	4	5	6	7	8	9	10	11	12	13	14	15	16	17	18	19	20	21	22	23	24	25	26	27	28	29	30	31
January	1	2	3	4	5	6	7	8	9	10	11	12	13	14	15	16	17	18	19	20	21	22	23	24	25	26	27	28	29	30	31
February	32	33	34	35	36	37	38	39	40	41	42	43	44	45	46	47	48	49	50	51	52	53	54	55	56	57	58	59			
March	60	61	62	63	64	65	66	67	68	69	70	71	72	73	74	75	76	77	78	79	80	81	82	83	84	85	86	87	88	89	90
April	91	92	93	94	95	96	97	98	99	100	101	102	103	104	105	106	107	108	109	110	111	112	113	114	115	116	117	118	119	120	
May	121	122	123	124	125	126	127	128	129	130	131	132	133	134	135	136	137	138	139	140	141	142	143	144	145	146	147	148	149	150	151
June	152	153	154	155	156	157	158	159	160	161	162	163	164	165	166	167	168	169	170	171	172	173	174	175	176	177	178	179	180	181	
July	182	183	184	185	186	187	188	189	190	191	192	193	194	195	196	197	198	199	200	201	202	203	204	205	206	207	208	209	210	211	212
August	213	214	215	216	217	218	219	220	221	222	223	224	225	226	227	228	229	230	231	232	233	234	235	236	237	238	239	240	241	242	243
September	244	245	246	247	248	249	250	251	252	253	254	255	256	257	258	259	260	261	262	263	264	265	266	267	268	269	270	271	272	273	
October	274	275	276	277	278	279	280	281	282	283	284	285	286	287	288	289	290	291	292	293	294	295	296	297	298	299	300	301	302	303	304
November	305	306	307	308	309	310	311	312	313	314	315	316	317	318	319	320	321	322	323	324	325	326	327	328	329	330	331	332	333	334	
December	335	336	337	338	339	340	341	342	343	344	345	346	347	348	349	350	351	352	353	354	355	356	357	358	359	360	361	362	363	364	365

Leap year from 1880 till present

18's	19's	20's
1880	1904	2000
1884	1908	2004
1888	1912	2008
1892	1916	2012
1896	1920	2016
	1924	2020
	1928	2024
	1932	
	1936	
	1940	
	1944	
	1948	
	1952	
	1956	
	1960	
	1964	
	1968	
	1972	
	1976	
	1980	
	1984	
	1988	
	1992	
	1996	

Now, with this tables above, let us assume the birthdate of someone to be 26th June 1992, and we plot the persons biorhythm chart for 29th November 2016. That being said that, at the later date he was 24 years old.

a) 20 × Number of days in a year; 20 × 365=7,300

4 × Number of days in a year; 4 × 365= 1,460

Then; 7,300 + 1460 =8,760(days)

b). From the year 1992 to 2016 we noticed that there were "6" leap years, so now, we add it to the number of days which we previously arrived at, now we get 8766(days).

C). Now, we go to the table of the year above, 26th June gives us 177, while 29th November gives us 333. So therefore, the subtraction of the two will give us 156. We can now add this to the given number of days (8766 + 156) =8922. Plus, one day, (which is the day in question) we arrive at 8923 days.

Cycle	Division	Remainder/ Biorhythm No
Physical(23)	8923 ÷ 23	22
Emotional(28)	8923 ÷ 28	19
Intellectual(33)	8923 ÷ 33	13

This calculations and chart represents the date 29 November only. But this diagram is just to give you a view and example of how the biorhythm chart is to be plotted, so you can easily make your own biogram for the month without the aid of an app. Yet, if you wish to go back in time, to see why you made a mistake on one occasion by failing to plan well, or you are trying to prepare yourself for a special future event, then, these simple calculations will help you on the way.

This simple arithmetic to Biorhythm provided in this book, can be done by anybody. If you do your calculations for the first day of any month, in order to arrive at the figures in each of the biorhythm cycles,

it would be easier to draw the curves, mark the critical days, and get the compatibility ratings, if comparing two biograms.

Bio rhythmically this would be a good day to make important decisions or write a test. But avoiding strenuous jobs and engaging only in routine task.

It is true that biorhythms are not magic and cannot predetermine your future, - like what you would become and or what you would do at a particular point in your life. But biorhythm will help you prepare yourself in advance against probabilities.

five

Late celebrities and their biorhythms

1. Leslie Nielsen: 11 February 1926 - 28th November 2010.

Biorhythm days= 30,971

Was treated for pneumonia, and his agent Kelly said he was fast asleep when he passed away. He was at peace with himself, he was in the positive phase Emotionally from the 26th to 28th but his physical and intellectual condition was in a critical phase, one on the 27th, the other on the 28th and his condition worsened during those periods.

2. George Orson Welles: 6 May 1915 - 10 October 1985

Biorhythm days = 25,725

He had been under treatment for both diabetes and heart ailment but in the night of his death, it was said that he was in high spirits which could be related to his physical state but just like his assistant coroner, Donald Messerle said, "he appears to die a natural death".

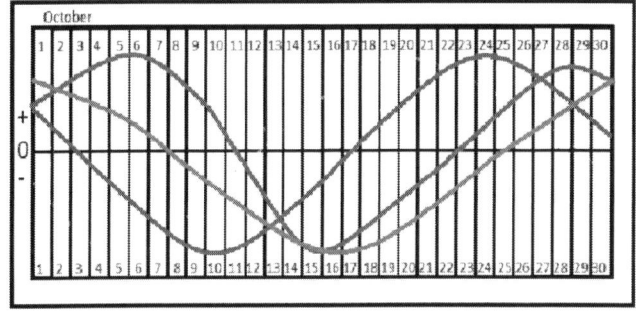

3. J. Edgar Hoover: 1 January 1895 - 2 May 1972

Biorhythm days= 28,247

He died in his sleep of a heart attack though he just crossed a physical critical stage a day before and he was in the negative phase emotionally and intellectually. Those three or two days before his death, was the best time for him to take good caution of himself.

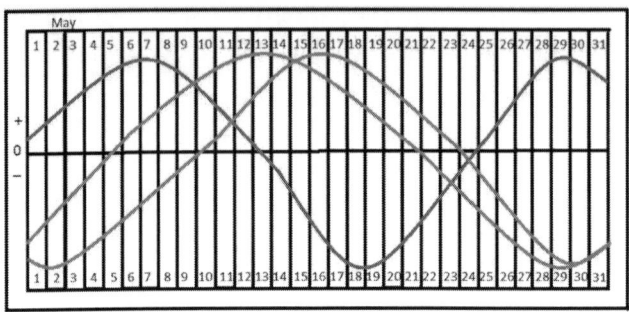

4. Celeste Holm: 29 April 1917 - 15 July 2012

Biorhythm days= 34,776

Holm had had different health complications in her life, which made her suffer and even to the point of retiring. But it was unfortunate she had to suffer an heart attack when all her bio- rhythms was in the negative phase. she could have had a chance of surviving if it were to be opposite. But her life was claimed on the 15th by an heart attack although all her rhythms was still in the negative phase, she had a double critical day both physically and emotionally the day she died.

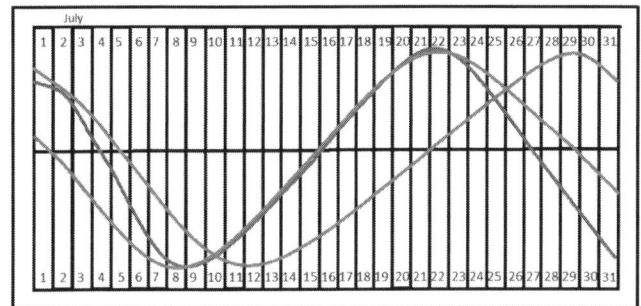

5. **Patrick. S. Wayne**: August 18 1952 - September 14 2009.

Biorhythm days= 20,846

In the late December 2007, after Swayze filmed the pilot episode for "*The beast*" he started to feel an unsettling pain down in his stomach so that three weeks after, he was diagnosed with pancreatic cancer. On the 21st of December 2007, Swayze was crossing a critical phase to the negative and he also had a critical day both on the 24th and 25th of that month

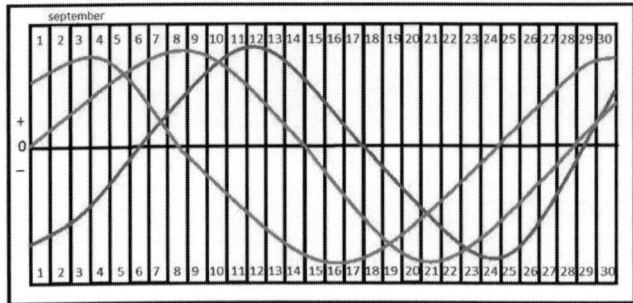

On march 5, 2008, Swayze was responding to treatment rapidly, at that time, he was going to the highest point in the physical positive rhythm and I'm sure that at 8th or 9th of that month, his immune system would be capable of standing any disease or infection to some extent which will make him feel that he isn't susceptible to the disease which is hunting him. At that point in time he was full of vigor.

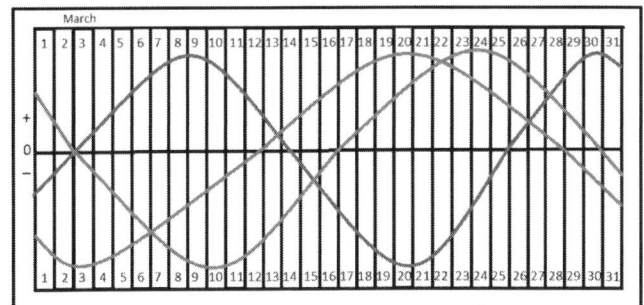

Swayze continued to live, with a positive and sound mind despite his disease and his self-will served him very well, in fact it could be said that he was lucky and his Biorhythms at those times, was in his favor. But on the 8th and 9th of January 2009, after crossing a physical critical stage, he was hospitalized with pneumonia. Maybe his immune system couldn't stand it any longer. He was discharged from the hospital on the 16th of that month, but yet, he wasn't still well.

Diagram:

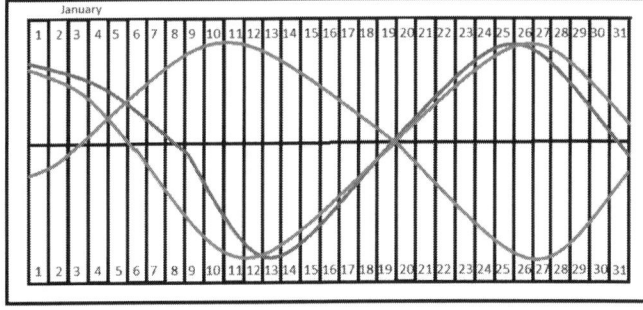

Despite that Swayze was a chronic smoker, he never resisted. And in August 2009, he was hospitalized for intestinal bleeding, this was his biorhythm for that month:

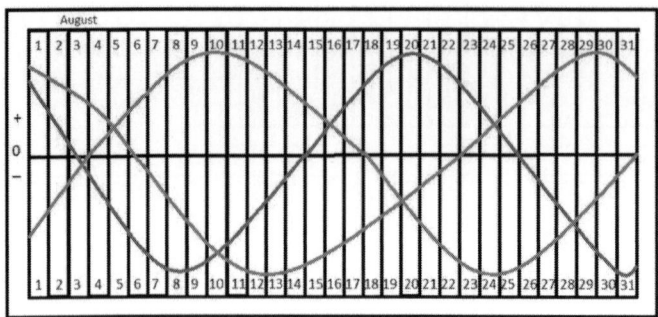

In September 14, 2009, Swayze died of pancreatic cancer. His physical condition was in his favor, but he was too tired of trying.

6. **Michael Jackson**: August 29, 1958 - 25 June 2007

Biorhythm days = 18,693

In fact, Jackson was in a good physical condition on the day before his death, and the day of his death. Arnold Klein, Jackson's dermatologist said, when he saw him at his office two days before his death, he was dancing for patients. This day should be day 23 in the biorhythm chart when he just crossed the critical phase to the physical positive phase, yet, he was intellectually positive. Ed Alonzo a magician at staples center had seen Jackson rehearsed for the Landen concert a night before his death, he said " Jackson looked great and had great energy. Autopsy report revealed that Jackson was still strong for his age, and that he had a sound heart. Although he had problem with his lungs but the cause of his death likely has more to do with abuse of drugs. Just like Klein said " Jackson misused prescription drugs" Just like the report said, Jackson died of acute Propofol and benzodiazepine intoxication, and it's inevitable.

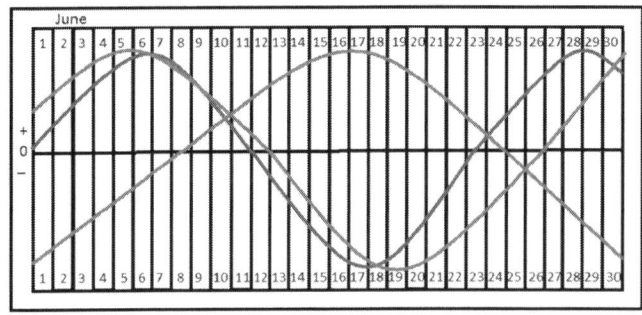

7. **Dennis Hopper**: 17 May 1936 - 29 May 2010

Biorhythm days= 27,040

Hopper was in a double critical stage a day before he was brought by an ambulance in a Manhattan hospital wearing an oxygen mask with numerous tubes all over, and he just crossed physical critical stage two days before.

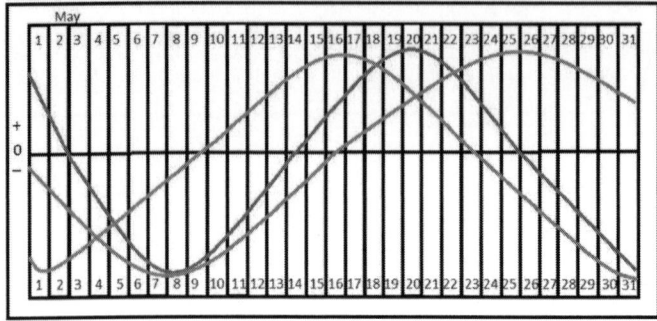

He was discharged on October 2 and then, all his three biorhythm cycles were on the positive phase, his physical cycle at the highest point.

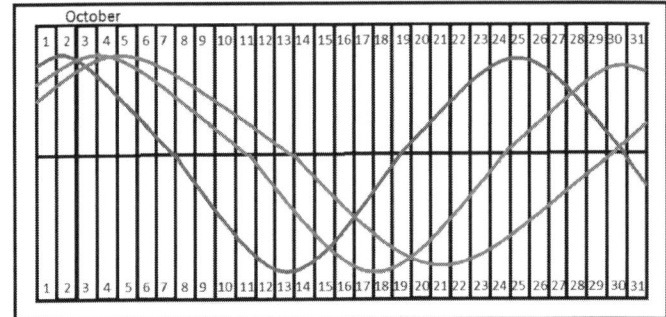

But by January 2010, it was reported that Dennis Hopper's cancer had metastasized to his bones.

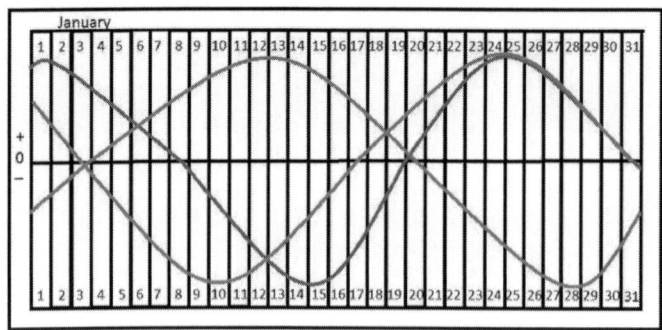

Hopper was terminally ill, and died of prostate cancer on the 29th of May 2010 when he was in the negative phase both physically and emotionally.

8. **Brittany Murphy:** November 10, 1977 - 20 December 2009

Biorhythm days = 11,728

Again, it was said that her death "appeared to be natural" and the primary cause of her death was pneumonia with secondary factors of iron deficiency anemia and multiple drug intoxication. Although, she was both in the negative phase both physically and emotionally at that particular date, the coroner stated that, she had been taking over the counter and prescription medications which contains "elevated levels" of hydrocodone, acetaminophen, Lb. Methamphetamine, and chlorpheniramine.

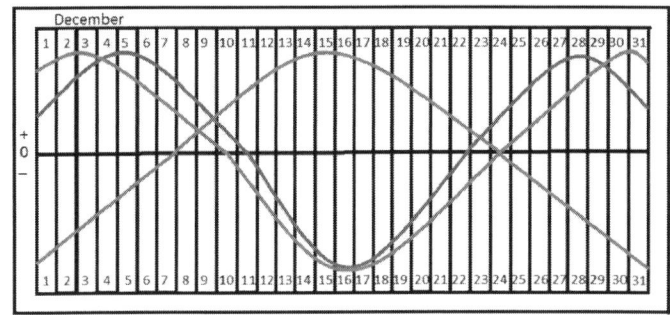

9. **Bernie Mac**: 3 October 1957 - 9 August 2008

Biorhythm days = 18,685

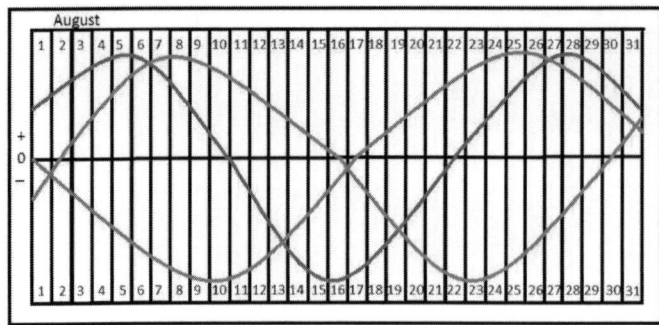

Bernard Jeffrey Mc collough had suffered from sarcoidosis. After a week of unsuccessful medical treatment, Mac died of complications of pneumonia, a day before a physical critical day.

10. **Health Ledger**: 4 April 1979 - 22 January 2008

Biorhythm days =10,665

Ledger death, has nothing to do with his biorhythm, it could also be said to be natural in nature, as with his biorhythm, he had more chance of surviving. He died of accidental overdose of prescription drugs.

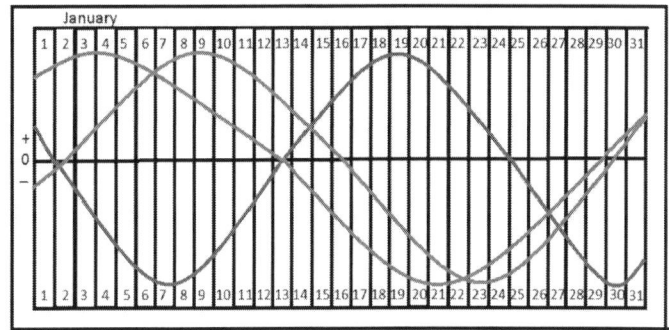

11. **Anna Nicole Smith**: 28 November 1967 - 8 February 2007

Biorhythm days = 11,728

Her death was somewhat similar to that of Health Ledger's. She was found dead in her hotel room in Florida. The cause of her death was due to accidental drug overdose of the sedative chloral hydrate combined with other prescription drugs in her system which contain (four benzodiazepines). A statement was made that the individual levels of any of the benzodiaphenes in her system would not have been sufficient to cause her death but high amount of chloride hydrate led to her overdose. But despite, she had a greater chance of surviving, as she had built more tolerance for the drug than the average person. Then we might look back at her biorhythm for that month and notice that she was in a physical critical day on the 8th. Is it likely that her tolerance for the drug at that date, failed her? Yes, its very likely as she could have taken more caution and the story might have been different.

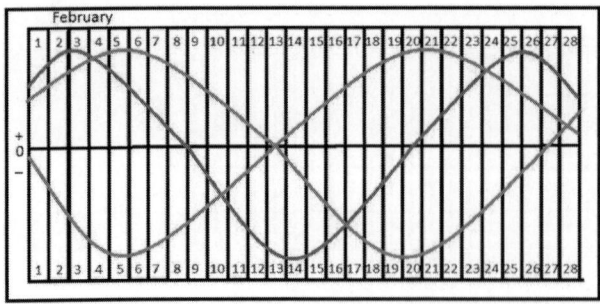

12. Steve Jobs: 24 February 1955 - 5 October 2011

Biorhythm days = 20,677

Steve jobs had previously been treated for islet-cell neuroendocrine pancreatic cancer which resulted in respiratory arrest. He lost consciousness on the 4th of October 2011 when he was in the physical and intellectual negative phase though he was in a good mood till the next day which he died, but he never had the strength to hold himself even if he was longing to meet the heavenly father.

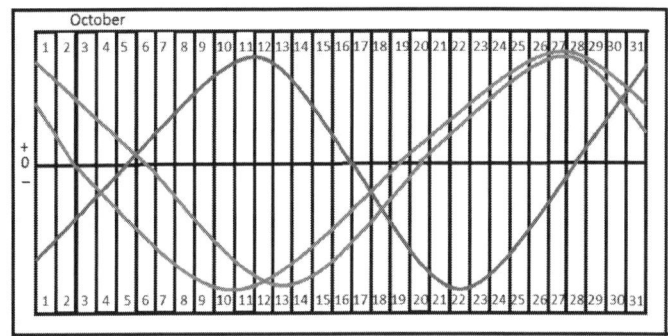

13. **David Bowie:** 8 January 1947 - 10 January 2016.

Biorhythm days = 25,205

Bowie died peacefully at least, his emotional biorhythm could say of that. He was at the lowest negative point the day he died of the long-battled cancer.

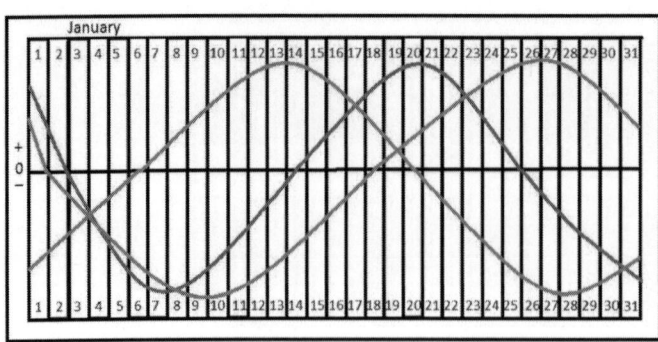

14. **Aaliyah**: 16 January 1979 - 25 August 2001

Biorhythm days = 8,257

She died in a Cessna 402B plane crash for the return trip back to Opa-locka airport in Florida. She couldn't have survived it anyways, she was in a physical critical day.

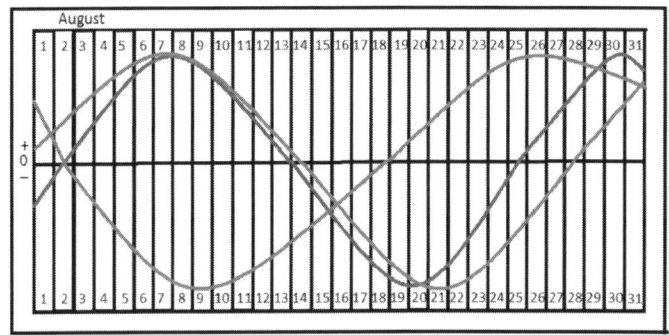

15. **Gene Wilder**: 11 June 1933 - 29 August 2016

Biorhythm days = 30,395

He kept the condition of his Alzheimer's disease private. He also died on a physical critical day.

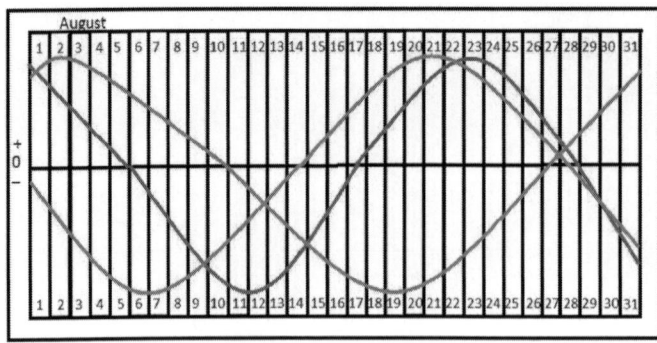

16. **Christopher Shannon Penn**: 10 October 1965 - 24 January   2006

Biorhythm days =15,234

Although, Penn was very used to drug taking, he died of cardiomyopathy which is a heart disease, which cause was discovered to be non- specific. He died when all his biorhythms were in the negative phase.

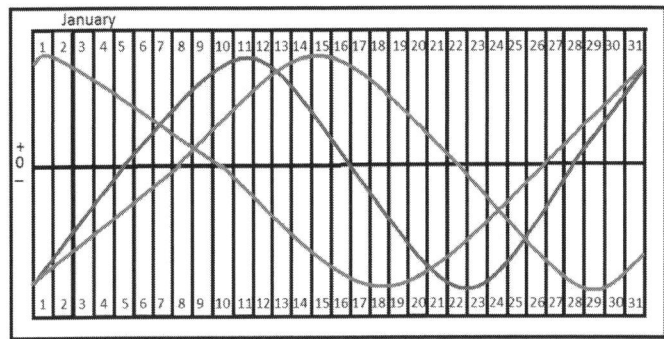

17. Brad Grey: 29 December 1957 - 14 May 2017

Biorhythm days= 22,144

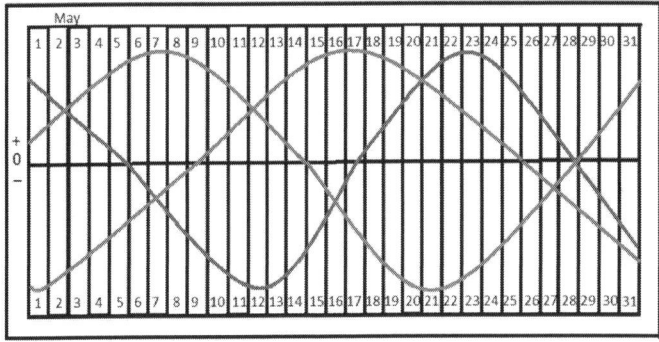

Bradgrey died of cancer beside his family at holmby hills. He should have taken careful watch, even if much could not be done. He was in a critical phase emotionally, positive intellectually, and negative physically

Six

Biorhythm and The Way of Life.

To every aspect of life, there is always a re-occurring rhythm like circles. These cycles are what keeps on going from time to time. It occurs in every aspect of life; biologically, spiritually, metaphysically, even from breathing, sleeping, waking and so on. These rhythms, even though the average man is not aware of it, affects every area and aspects of his life until he dies. When he is asleep, it affects his subconscious, since every man when asleep, is half conscious.

Biorhythm affects a man's behavioral pattern, and it determines his actions to some extent. Biorhythms can be used as a practical purpose for anticipating potential danger or success in the nearest future. So many Japanese use this, to anticipate forthcoming danger days, in industrial occupations, especially their transportation network and this has reduced their accident rate to some extent. knowing that you are likely to be intellectually down on the examination day, may allow you to postpone it till you are ready. Some Clinics I know, make use of the Biorhythms and some do not even make use of it at all. But I strongly suggest that biorhythm be introduced to all physicians, especially the ones who specializes in surgery. You know, if the physician consults the patients biogram and study the next critical stage of that patient, he would pay special attention by making sure the patient is in a good condition at that moment.

Any athlete or driver who doesn't know about biorhythms is missing out on a lot. Reasons for too many accidents and injuries. A car racer who drives on a day when he is on the critical stage, physically and emotionally, he got too sentimental just because the other dude overtook him, is taking on a greater risk; he might get himself in the hospital bed before he even realizes it and as long as biorhythm is concerned, it applies to pilots, bus drivers, and in general, those involved in transportation.

In a car crash, some people died, some survived - This also has a lot to do with biorhythms. The heavy weight champion, our friend Mohammad Ali got his jaw broken in a fight with Newton Ken. Mohammad Ali's biorhythm shows that he was on a double critical phase on that day.

I've heard of events whereby, famous public speakers lost their lines, when addressing their audience, but quickly they made up ways to cover the embarrassment. If they had known they were in the intellectual critical day, they could have saved themselves those embarrassment by careful preparations and avoiding being over-confident.

Funny enough, A mathematics teacher could not remember the formula for calculating the area of a sector until he cunningly asked his pupils as he was unsure - he was double critical phase that day, one of which was intellectual. I know of a couple that agreed to consider implementing biorhythms in their daily life; not that they really believed in it, but they partially believed in the theory of cyclic performance, and since they desperately wanted to improve their marital life, they considered biorhythms out of curiosity. Later, they were like "Biorhythms had made us understand our differences.... we made compromises".

So, you might have been wandering, why am I not getting along with this guy, or why is there always a misunderstanding between us, check your biorhythms each, you would find the answers.

Humans are natural diurnal creatures. Our body temperature reaches a peak in the morning hours at about 7:00a.m to 9: 00a.m, but at its lowest when we are asleep. But some people are the opposite though they are rare - This makes us partially divided into the "morning people" and "evening people". It is very strange that some are more vibrant during the evening period and this is common among those, engaged in night shift work. Since they have been accustomed to working nights, their body system naturally adapts to the changes. To them, the evening periods seems an "Ignition to life".

If a stage in your biorhythm cycle, is similar to that of your partner's then there is likely a chance that you will behave similarly in that particular pattern. That is; a cyclic performance happening at the same time.

Funny enough, the fact that everything pertaining to life, happens in cycles, can be said of trends, especially fashion- reoccurring trends. But the question now is, can we predetermine our exact actions through means, just like biorhythm? Maybe, maybe not, depending on the level of discovery in this rapid growing age but all I can proudly say now is that it gives you informed judgement of a situation.

The secrets of rhythms and cycles have been uncovered for more than the past twenty decades through various scientists and they testify that we go through certain rhythmical pattern over and over again. Our body cells, replaces itself after dead cells are gone, we feel like we are still the same as we are a day before but, we grow every day. Our mental faculty expands because of the new things we learn, as we sleep, our hairs and nails grow and the average man eats 1,095 times a year, yet his stomach never stops to demand for food nor his mouth tired of chewing. In the early mornings, you seem to grow half an inch taller later in that same morning, you shrink back. These are cyclic performances executing their role.

Early waking hours and late evening hours are the periods when we are more vibrant intellectually. The brain works faster and smarter than mid-days. Try to do a study late at night, then revise on it earliest in the morning, you would be surprised at how you would assimilate without difficulty and this also is due to your temperature during this period, all this, a form of cellular replacement cycle.

Our brain functions in cycles, even the ability to remember. Sometimes, we seem to forget even the simplest things. This is only natural depending on the individual but yet still a form of cellular replacement cycle. The earth rotates in circles, the repeated alternation of night and day, another cyclic performance or is it a coincidence? Even magic, involves the use of cyclic performance. The force of cycles and rhythms is what holds the earth together and if it is missing, there is going to be a resounding chaos.

Has the duration of the day ever shifted from the usual 24hours or have you ever experienced continuous darkness for a whole day apart from the eclipse of the sun? Right from the former days hitherto, there had always been some complications in understanding the principles involving cycles. We do not understand the meaning of this rhythm all around us. but one day, we shall find the answers to our underlying inquisition.

Printed in Great Britain
by Amazon